A Beginners \

Recipe Book

Discover the Benefits of Eating Well

with Vegan Recipes, Lose Weight

Fast, Energize your Body and

Improve your Well-Being

Franck Renner

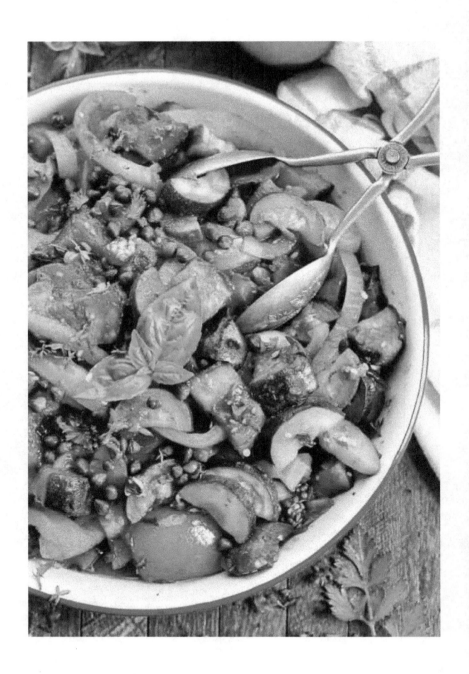

Table of Contents

INTRODUCTION

The Merriam Webster Dictionary defines a vegetarian as one contains a wholly of vegetables, grains, nuts, fruits, and sometimes eggs or dairy products. It has also been described as a plant-based diet that relies wholly on plant-foods such as fruits, whole grains, herbs, vegetables, nuts, seeds, and spices. Whatever way you want to look at it, the reliance wholly on plants stands the vegetarian diet out from other types of diets. People become vegetarians for different reasons. Some take up this nutritional plan for medical or health reasons. For example, people suffering from cardiovascular diseases or who stand the risk of developing such diseases are usually advised to refrain from meat generally and focus on a plant-based diet, rich in fruits and vegetables. Some other individuals become vegetarians for religious or ethical reasons.

On this side of the spectrum are Hinduism, Jainism, Buddhism, Seventh-Day Adventists, and some other religions. It is believed that being a vegetarian is part of being holy and keeping with the ideals of non-violence. For ethical reasons, some animal rights activists are also vegetarians based on the belief that animals have rights and should not be slaughtered for food. Yet another set of persons become vegetarians based on food preference. Such individuals are naturally more disposed to a plant-based diet and find meat and other related food products less pleasurable. Some refrain from meat as a protest against climate change. This is based on the environmental concern that rearing livestock contributes to climate change and greenhouse gas emissions and the waste of natural resources in maintaining such livestock. People are usually very quick to throw words around without exactly knowing what a Vegetarian Diet means. In the same vein, the term "vegetarian" has become a popular one in recent years. What exactly does this word connote, and what does it not mean?

At its simplest, the word "vegetarian" refers to a person who refrains from eating meat, beef, pork, lard, chicken, or even fish. Depending on the kind of vegetarian it is, however, a vegetarian could either eat or exclude from his diet animal products. Animal products would refer to foods such as eggs, dairy products, and even honey! A vegetarian diet would, therefore, refer to the nutritional plan of the void of meat. It is the eating lifestyle of individuals who depend on plant-based foods for nutrition. It excludes animal products, particularly meat - a common denominator for all kinds of Vegetarians - from their diets. A vegetarian could also be defined as a meal plan that consists of foods coming majorly from plants to the exclusion of meat, poultry, and seafood.

This kind of Vegetarian diet usually contains no animal protein.

It is completely understandable from the discussion so far that the term "vegetarian" is more or less a blanket term covering different plant-based diets. While reliance majorly on plant foods is consistent in all the different types of vegetarians, they have some underlying differences. The different types of vegetarians are discussed below:

Veganism: This is undoubtedly the strictest type of vegetarian diet. Vegans exclude the any animal product. It goes as far as avoiding animal-derived ingredients contained in processed foods. Whether its meat, poultry products like eggs, dairy products inclusive of milk, honey, or even gelatin, they all are excluded from the vegans.

Some vegans go beyond nutrition and go as far as refusing to wear clothes that contain animal products. This means such vegans do not wear leather, wool, or silk.

Lacto-vegetarian: This kind of vegetarian excludes meat, fish, and poultry. However, it allows the inclusion of dairy products such as milk, yogurt, cheese, and butter. The hint is perhaps in the name since Lacto means milk in Latin.

Ovo-Vegetarian: Meat and dairy products are excluded under this diet, but eggs could be consumed. Ovo means egg.

Lacto-Ovo Vegetarian: This appears to be the hybrid of the Ovo Vegetarian and the Lacto-Vegetarian. This is the most famous type of vegetarian diet and is usually what comes to mind when people think of the Vegetarian. This type of Vegetarian bars all kinds of meat but allows for the consumption of eggs and dairy products.

Pollotarian: This vegetarian allows the consumption of chicken.

Pescatarian: This refers to the vegetarian that consumes fish. More people are beginning to subscribe to this kind of diet due to health reasons.

Flexitarian: Flexitarians are individuals who prefer plant-based foods to meat but have no problem eating meats once in a while. They are also referred to as semi-vegetarians.

Raw Vegan: This is also called the raw food and consists of a vegan that is yet to be processed and has also not been heated over 46 C. This kind of diet has its root in the belief that nutrients and minerals present in the plant diet are lost when cooked on temperature above 46 C and could also become harmful to the body.

Lime in the Coconut Chia Pudding

Preparation Time: 10 minutes

Cooking Time: 20 minutes

Servings: 4

Ingredients:

- Zest and juice of 1 lime
- 1 (14-ounce) can coconut milk
- 1 to 2 dates, or 1 tablespoon coconut or other unrefined sugar, or 1 tablespoon maple syrup, or 10 to 15 drops pure liquid stevia
- 2 tablespoons chia seeds, whole or ground
- 2 teaspoons matcha green tea powder (optional)

Directions:

1. Preparing the Ingredients.
2. Blend all the ingredients in a blender until smooth. Chill in the fridge for about 20 minutes, then serve topped with one or more of the topping ideas.
3. Try blueberries, blackberries, sliced strawberries, Coconut Whipped Cream, or toasted unsweetened coconut.

Nutrition: Calories 381 Fat 17.1 g Carbohydrates 4.1 g Sugar 0.6 g Protein 50.6 g Cholesterol 358 mg

Mint Chocolate Chip Sorbet

Preparation Time: 5 minutes

Cooking Time: 0 minute

Servings: 1

Ingredients:

- 1 frozen banana
- 1 tablespoon almond butter, or peanut butter, or other nut or seed butter
- 2 tablespoons fresh mint, minced
- ¼ cup or less non-dairy milk (only if needed)
- 2 to 3 tablespoons non-dairy chocolate chips, or cocoa nibs
- 2 to 3 tablespoons goji berries (optional)

Directions:

1. Preparing the Ingredients.
2. Put the banana, almond butter, and mint in a food processor or blender and purée until smooth.
3. Add the non-dairy milk if needed to keep blending (but only if needed, as this will make the texture less solid). Pulse the chocolate chips

and goji berries (if using) into the mix so they're roughly chopped up.

Nutrition: Calories 299 Fat 16 g Carbohydrates 3 g Sugar 6 g Protein 38 g Cholesterol 108 mg

Peach-Mango Crumble (Pressure cooker)

Preparation Time: 10 minutes

Cooking Time: 6 minutes

Servings: 4-6

Ingredient:

- 3 cups chopped fresh or frozen peaches
- 3 cups chopped fresh or frozen mangos
- 4 tablespoons unrefined sugar or pure maple syrup, divided
- 1 cup gluten-free rolled oats
- ½ cup shredded coconut, sweetened or unsweetened
- 2 tablespoons coconut oil or vegan margarine

Directions:

1. Preparing the Ingredients. In a 6- to 7-inch round baking dish, toss together the peaches, mangos, and 2 tablespoons of sugar. In a food processor, combine the oats, coconut, coconut oil, and remaining 2 tablespoons of sugar. Pulse until combined. (If you use maple syrup, you'll

need less coconut oil. Start with just the syrup and add oil if the mixture isn't sticking together.) Sprinkle the oat mixture over the fruit mixture.

2. Cover the dish with aluminum foil. Put a trivet in the bottom of your electric pressure cooker's cooking pot and pour in a cup or two of water. Using a foil sling or silicone helper handles, lower the pan onto the trivet.

3. High pressure for 6 minutes. Close and lock the lid, and select High Pressure for 6 minutes.

4. Pressure Release. Once the **Cooking Time:** is complete, quick release the pressure. Unlock and remove the lid.

5. Let cool for a few minutes before carefully lifting out the dish with oven mitts or tongs. Scoop out portions to serve.

Nutrition: Calories 275 Fat 19 g Carbohydrates 19 g Sugar 4 g Protein 14 g Cholesterol 60 mg

Zesty Orange-Cranberry Energy Bites

Preparation Time: 10 minutes

Cooking Time: 15 minutes

Servings: 12

Ingredients:

- 2 tablespoons almond butter, or cashew or sunflower seed butter
- 2 tablespoons maple syrup, or brown rice syrup
- ¾ cup cooked quinoa
- ¼ cup sesame seeds, toasted
- 1 tablespoon chia seeds
- ½ teaspoon almond extract, or vanilla extract
- Zest of 1 orange
- 1 tablespoon dried cranberries
- ¼ cup ground almonds

Directions:

1. Preparing the Ingredients.
2. In a medium bowl, mix together the nut or seed butter and syrup until smooth and creamy. Stir in the rest of the ingredients, and mix to make

---

23

sure the consistency is holding together in a ball. Form the mix into 12 balls.

3. Place them on a baking sheet lined with parchment or waxed paper and put in the fridge to set for about 15 minutes.

4. If your balls aren't holding together, it's likely because of the moisture content of your cooked quinoa. Add more nut or seed butter mixed with syrup until it all sticks together.

Nutrition: Calories 493 Fat 33 g Carbohydrates 8 g Sugar 9 g Protein 47 g Cholesterol 135 mg

Almond-Date Energy Bites

Preparation Time: 5 minutes

Cooking Time: 15 minutes

Servings: 24

Ingredients:

- 1 cup dates, pitted
- 1 cup unsweetened shredded coconut
- ¼ cup chia seeds
- ¾ cup ground almonds
- ¼ cup cocoa nibs, or non-dairy chocolate chips

Directions:

1. Purée everything in a food processor until crumbly and sticking together, pushing down the sides whenever necessary to keep it blending. If you don't have a food processor, you can mash soft Medjool dates. But if you're using harder baking dates, you'll have to soak them and then try to purée them in a blender.
2. Form the mix into 24 balls and place them on a baking sheet lined with parchment or waxed paper. Put in the fridge to set for about 15

minutes. Use the softest dates you can find. Medjool dates are the best for this purpose. The hard dates you see in the baking aisle of your supermarket are going to take a long time to blend up. If you use those, try soaking them in water for at least an hour before you start, and then draining.

Nutrition: Calories 171 Fat 4 g Carbohydrates 7 g Sugar 7 g Protein 22 g Cholesterol 65 mg

Pumpkin Pie Cups (Pressure cooker)

Preparation Time: 5 minutes

Cooking Time: 6 minutes

Servings: 4-6

Ingredients:

- 1 cup canned pumpkin purée
- 1 cup nondairy milk
- 6 tablespoons unrefined sugar or pure maple syrup (less if using sweetened milk), plus more for sprinkling
- ¼ cup spelt flour or whole-grain flour
- ½ teaspoon pumpkin pie spice
- Pinch salt

Directions:

1. Preparing the Ingredients. In a medium bowl, stir together the pumpkin, milk, sugar, flour, pumpkin pie spice, and salt. Pour the mixture into 4 heat-proof ramekins. Sprinkle a bit more sugar on the top of each, if you like. Put a trivet in the bottom of your electric pressure cooker's

cooking pot and pour in a cup or two of water. Place the ramekins onto the trivet, stacking them if needed (3 on the bottom, 1 on top).

2. High pressure for 6 minutes. Close and lock the lid, and select High Pressure for 6 minutes.

3. Pressure Release. Once the **Cooking Time:** is complete, quick release the pressure. Unlock and remove the lid. Let cool for a few minutes before carefully lifting out the ramekins with oven mitts or tongs. Let cool for at least 10 minutes before serving.

Nutrition: Calories 152 Fat 4 g Carbohydrates 4 g Sugar 8 g Protein 18 g Cholesterol 51 mg

Coconut and Almond Truffles

Preparation Time: 15 minutes

Cooking Time: 0 minutes

Servings: 8

Ingredients:

- 1 cup pitted dates
- 1 cup almonds
- ½ cup sweetened cocoa powder, plus extra for coating
- ½ cup unsweetened shredded coconut
- ¼ cup pure maple syrup
- 1 teaspoon vanilla extract
- 1 teaspoon almond extract
- ¼ teaspoon sea salt

Directions:

1. Preparing the Ingredients.
2. In the bowl of a food processor, combine all the ingredients and process until smooth. Chill the mixture for about 1 hour.
3. Roll the mixture into balls and then roll the balls in cocoa powder to coat.

4. Serve immediately or keep chilled until ready to serve.

Nutrition: Calories 126 Fat 5 g Carbohydrates 13 g Sugar 7 g Protein 5 g Cholesterol 0 mg

Fudgy Brownies (Pressure cooker)

Preparation Time: 10 minutes

Cooking Time: 5 minutes

Servings: 4-6

Ingredients:

- 3 ounces dairy-free dark chocolate
- 1 tablespoon coconut oil or vegan margarine
- ½ cup applesauce
- 2 tablespoons unrefined sugar
- 1/3 cup whole-grain flour
- ½ teaspoon baking powder
- Pinch salt

Directions:

1. Preparing the Ingredients. Put a trivet in your electric pressure cooker's cooking pot and pour in a cup or two of two of water. Select Sauté or Simmer. In a large heat-proof glass or ceramic bowl, combine the chocolate and coconut oil. Place the bowl over the top of your pressure cooker, as you would a double boiler. Stir

occasionally until the chocolate is melted, then turn off the pressure cooker. Stir the applesauce and sugar into the chocolate mixture. Add the flour, baking powder, and salt and stir just until combined. Pour the batter into 3 heat-proof ramekins. Put them in a heat-proof dish and cover with aluminum foil. Using a foil sling or silicone helper handles, lower the dish onto the trivet. (Alternately, cover each ramekin with foil and place them directly on the trivet, without the dish.)

2. High pressure for 6 minutes. Close and lock the lid, and select High Pressure for 5 minutes.

3. Pressure Release. Once the **Cooking Time:** is complete, quick release the pressure. Unlock and remove the lid.

4. Let cool for a few minutes before carefully lifting out the dish, or ramekins, with oven mitts or tongs. Let cool for a few minutes more before serving.

5. Top with fresh raspberries and an extra drizzle of melted chocolate.

Nutrition: Calories 256 Fat 29 g Carbohydrates 1 g Sugar 0.5 g Protein 11 g Cholesterol 84 mg

Chocolate Macaroons

Preparation Time: 10 minutes

Cooking Time: 15 minutes

Servings: 8

Ingredients:

- 1 cup unsweetened shredded coconut
- 2 tablespoons cocoa powder
- 2/3 cup coconut milk
- ¼ cup agave
- pinch of sea salt

Directions:

1. Preparing the Ingredients.
2. Preheat the oven to 350°F. Line a baking sheet with parchment paper. In a medium saucepan, cook all the ingredients over -medium-high heat until a firm dough is formed. Scoop the dough into balls and place on the baking sheet.
3. Bake for 15 minutes, remove from the oven, and let cool on the baking sheet.
4. Serve cooled macaroons or store in a tightly sealed container for up to

Nutrition: Calories 371 Fat 15 g Carbohydrates 7 g Sugar 2 g Protein 41 g Cholesterol 135 mg

Express Coconut Flax Pudding

Preparation Time: 5 minutes

Cooking Time: 15 minutes

Servings: 4

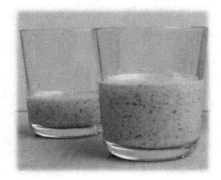

Ingredients:

- 1 Tbsp. coconut oil softened
- 1 Tbsp. coconut cream
- 2 cups coconut milk canned
- 3/4 cup ground flax seed
- 4 Tbsp. coconut palm sugar (or to taste)

Directions:

1. Press SAUTÉ button on your Instant Pot
2. Add coconut oil, coconut cream, coconut milk, and ground flaxseed.
3. Stir about 5 - 10 minutes.

4. Lock lid into place and set on the MANUAL setting for 5 minutes.

5. When the timer beeps, press "Cancel" and carefully flip the Quick Release valve to let the pressure out.

6. Add the palm sugar and stir well.

7. Taste and adjust sugar to taste.

8. Allow pudding to cool down completely.

9. Place the pudding in an airtight container and refrigerate for up to 2 weeks.

Nutrition: Calories: 140 Fat: 2g Fiber: 23g Carbs: 22g Protein: 47g

Full-flavored Vanilla Ice Cream

Preparation Time: 5 minutes

Cooking Time: 20 minutes

Servings: 8

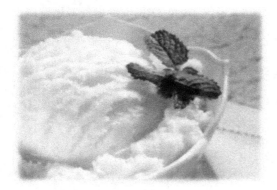

Ingredients:

- 1 1/2 cups canned coconut milk
- 1 cup coconut whipping cream
- 1 frozen banana cut into chunks
- 1 cup vanilla sugar
- 3 Tbsp. apple sauce
- 2 tsp pure vanilla extract
- 1 tsp Xanthan gum or agar-agar thickening agent

Directions:

1. Add all ingredients in a food processor; process until all ingredients combined well.

2. Place the ice cream mixture in a freezer-safe container with a lid over.

3. Freeze for at least 4 hours.

4. Remove frozen mixture to a bowl and beat with a mixer to break up the ice crystals.

5. Repeat this process 3 to 4 times.

6. Let the ice cream at room temperature for 15 minutes before serving.

Nutrition: Calories: 342 Fat: 15g Fiber: 11g Carbs: 8g Protein: 10g

Irresistible Peanut Cookies

Preparation Time: 5 minutes

Cooking Time: 25 minutes

Servings: 8

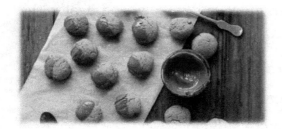

Ingredients:

- 4 Tbsp. all-purpose flour
- 1 tsp baking soda
- pinch of salt
- 1/3 cup granulated sugar
- 1/3 cup peanut butter softened
- 3 Tbsp. applesauce
- 1/2 tsp pure vanilla extract

Directions:

1. Preheat oven to 350 F.
2. Combine the flour, baking soda, salt, and sugar in a mixing bowl; stir.

3. Add all remaining ingredients and stir well to form a dough.

4. Roll dough into cookie balls/patties.

5. Arrange your cookies onto greased (with oil or cooking spray) baking sheet.

6. Bake for about 8 to 10 minutes.

7. Let cool for at least 15 minutes before removing from tray.

8. Remove cookies from the tray and let cool completely.

9. Place your peanut butter cookies in an airtight container, and keep refrigerated up to 10 days.

Nutrition: Calories: 211 Fat: 18g Fiber: 20g Carbs: 17g Protein: 39g

Murky Almond Cookies

Preparation Time: 10 minutes

Cooking Time: 15 minutes

Servings: 12

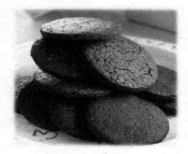

Ingredients:

- 4 Tbsp. cocoa powder
- 2 cups almond flour
- 1/4 tsp salt
- 1/2 tsp baking soda
- 5 Tbsp. coconut oil melted
- 2 Tbsp. almond milk
- 1 1/2 tsp almond extract
- 1 tsp vanilla extract
- 4 Tbsp. corn syrup or honey

Directions:

1. Preheat oven to 340 F degrees.

2. Grease a large baking sheet; set aside.

3. Combine the cocoa powder, almond flour, salt, and baking soda in a bowl.

4. In a separate bowl, whisk melted coconut oil, almond milk, almond and vanilla extract, and corn syrup or honey.

5. Combine the almond flour mixture with the almond milk mixture and stir until all ingredients incorporate well.

6. Roll tablespoons of the dough into balls, and arrange onto a prepared baking sheet.

7. Bake for 12 to 15 minutes.

8. Remove from the oven and transfer onto a plate lined with a paper towel.

9. Allow cookies to cool down completely and store in an airtight container at room temperature for about four days.

Nutrition: Calories: 508 Fat: 12g Fiber: 9g Carbs: 24g Protein: 40g

Orange Semolina Halva

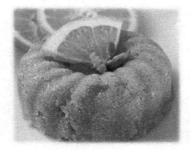

Preparation Time: 15 minutes

Cooking Time: 5 minutes

Servings: 12

Ingredients:

- 6 cups fresh orange juice
- Zest from 3 oranges
- 3 cups brown sugar
- 1 1/4 cup semolina flour
- 1 Tbsp. almond butter (plain, unsalted)
- 4 Tbsp. ground almond
- 1/4 tsp cinnamon

Directions:

1. Heat the orange juice, orange zest with brown sugar in a pot.
2. Stir over medium heat until sugar is dissolved.

---

3. Add the semolina flour and cook over low heat for 15 minutes; stir occasionally.

4. Add almond butter, ground almonds, and cinnamon, and stir well.

5. Cook, frequently stirring, for further 5 minutes.

6. Transfer the halva mixture into a mold, let it cool and refrigerate for at least 4 hours.

7. Keep refrigerated in a sealed container for one week.

Nutrition: Calories: 285 Fat: 28g Fiber: 7g Carbs: 34g Protein: 23g

Seasoned Cinnamon Mango Popsicles

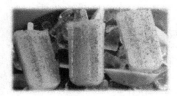

Preparation Time: 15 minutes

Cooking Time: 0 minute

Servings: 6

Ingredients:

- 1 1/2 cups of mango pulp
- 1 mango cut in cubes
- 1 cup brown sugar (packed)
- 2 Tbsp. lemon juice freshly squeezed
- 1 tsp cinnamon
- 1 pinch of salt

Directions:

1. Add all ingredients into your blender.
2. Blend until brown sugar dissolved.
3. Pour the mango mixture evenly in popsicle molds or cups.
4. Insert sticks into each mold.

5. Place molds in a freezer, and freeze for at least 5 to 6 hours.

6. Before serving, un-mold easy your popsicles placing molds under lukewarm water.

Nutrition: Calories: 423 Fat: 2g Fiber: 0g Carbs: 20g Protein: 33g

Strawberry Molasses Ice Cream

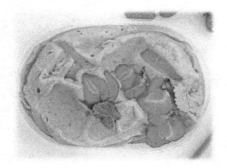

Preparation Time: 20 minutes

Cooking Time: 0 minute

Servings: 8

Ingredients:

- 1 lb. strawberries
- 3/4 cup coconut palm sugar (or granulated sugar)
- 1 cup coconut cream
- 1 Tbsp. molasses
- 1 tsp balsamic vinegar
- 1/2 tsp agar-agar
- 1/2 tsp pure strawberry extract

Directions:

1. Add strawberries, date sugar, and the balsamic vinegar in a blender; blend until completely combined.
2. Place the mixture in the refrigerator for one hour.
3. In a mixing bowl, beat the coconut cream with an electric mixer to make a thick mixture.
4. Add molasses, balsamic vinegar, agar-agar, and beat for further one minute or until combined well.
5. Keep frozen in a freezer-safe container (with plastic film and lid over).

Nutrition: Calories: 110 Fat: 31g Fiber: 18g Carbs: 15g Protein: 12g

Strawberry-Mint Sorbet

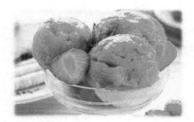

Preparation Time: 10 minutes

Cooking Time: 5 minutes

Servings: 6

Ingredients:

- 1 cup of granulated sugar
- 1 cup of orange juice
- 1 lb. frozen strawberries
- 1 tsp pure peppermint extract

Directions:

1. Add sugar and orange juice in a saucepan.
2. Stir over high heat and boil for 5 minutes or until sugar dissolves.
3. Remove from the heat and let it cool down.
4. Add strawberries into a blender, and blend until smooth.

5. Pour syrup into strawberries, add peppermint extract and stir until all ingredients combined well.

6. Transfer mixture to a storage container, cover tightly, and freeze until ready to serve.

Nutrition: Calories: 257 Fat: 13g Fiber: 37g Carbs: 11g Protein: 8g

Keto Chocolate Brownies

Preparation Time: 15 minutes

Cooking Time: 15 minutes

Servings: 4

Ingredients:

- ¼ t. of the following:
- salt
- baking soda
- ½ c. of the following:
- sweetener of your choice
- coconut flour
- vegetable oil
- water
- ¼ c. of the following:
- cocoa powder
- almond milk yogurt
- 1 tbsp. ground flax
- 1 t. vanilla extract

Directions:

1. Bring the oven to 350 heat setting.

2. Mix the ground flax, vanilla, yogurt, oil, and water; set to the side for 10 minutes.

3. Line an oven-safe 8x8 baking dish with parchment paper.

4. After 10 minutes have passed, add coconut flour, cocoa powder, sweetener, baking soda, and salt.

5. Bake for 15 minutes; make sure that you placed it in the center. When they come out, they will look underdone.

6. Place in the refrigerator and let them firm up overnight.

Nutrition: Calories: 208 Fat: 3g Fiber: 4g Carbs: 7g Protein: 27g

Chocolate Fat Bomb

Preparation Time: 5 minutes

Cooking Time: 0 minutes

Servings: 14

Ingredients:

- 1 tbsp. liquid sweetener of your choice.
- ¼ c. of the following:
- coconut oil, melted
- cocoa powder
- ½ c. almond butter

Directions:

1. Mix the ingredients in a medium bowl until smooth. Pour into the candy molds or ice cube trays.
2. Put in the freezer to set.
3. Store in freezer.

Nutrition: Calories: 241 Fat: 2g Fiber: 16g Carbs: 9g Protein: 22g

Vanilla Cheesecake

Preparation Time: 3 hours 20 minutes

Cooking Time: 0 minute

Servings: 10

Ingredients:

- 1 tbsp. vanilla extract,
- 2 ½ tbsp. lemon juice
- ½ c. coconut oil
- 1/8 t. stevia powder
- 6 tbsp. coconut milk
- 1 ½ c. blanched almonds soaked

Crust:

- 2 tbsp. coconut oil
- 1 ½ c. almonds

Directions:

For the Crust:

1. In a food processor, add the almonds and coconut oil and pulse until crumbles start to form.
2. Line a 7-inch springform pan with parchment paper and firmly press the crust into the bottom.

3. For the Sauce:

4. Bring a saucepan of water to a boil and soak the almonds for 2 hours. Drain and shake to dry.

5. Next, add the almonds to the food processor and blend until completely smooth.

6. Add vanilla, lemon, coconut oil, stevia, and coconut milk and blend until smooth.

7. Pour over the crust and freeze overnight or for a minimum of 3 hours.

8. Serve and enjoy.

Nutrition: Calories: 267 Fat: 13g Fiber: 14g Carbs: 17g Protein: 10g

Chocolate Mousse

Preparation Time: 5 minutes

Cooking Time: 0 minute

Servings: 2

Ingredients:

- 6 drops liquid stevia extract
- ½ t. cinnamon
- 3 tbsp. cocoa powder, unsweetened
- 1 c. coconut milk

Directions:

1. On the day before, place the coconut milk into the refrigerator overnight.
2. Remove the coconut milk from the refrigerator; it should be very thick.
3. Whisk in cocoa powder with an electric mixer.
4. Add stevia and cinnamon and whip until combined.
5. Place in individual bowls and serve and enjoy.

Nutrition: Calories: 130 Fat: 5g Fiber: 3g Carbs: 6g Protein: 7g

OTHER RECIPES

Tahini Miso Dressing

Preparation Time: 10 minutes

Cooking Time: 0 minute

Servings: 2

Ingredients:

- ¼ cup tahini
- 1 tablespoon tamari or low-sodium soy sauce
- 1 tablespoon white miso
- 1 tablespoon freshly squeezed lemon juice
- 1 tablespoon maple syrup or honey
- ¼ cup warm water
- Freshly ground black pepper

Directions:

1. In a small bowl, whisk the tahini, tamari, miso, lemon juice, and maple syrup together. Whisk in the water and black pepper. Store in an airtight container in the refrigerator for up to six months.

Nutrition: Calories: 76 Fat: 6g Carbs: 5g Protein: 2g

Balsamic Roasted Tomatoes

Preparation Time: 10 minutes

Cooking Time: 4 hours

Servings: 6

Ingredients:

- 6 medium tomatoes or 1 pint cherry tomatoes
- ¼ cup, plus 1 tablespoon olive oil
- Kosher salt
- Freshly ground black pepper
- 2 teaspoons balsamic vinegar

Directions:

1. Preheat the oven to 300°F. Put your rimmed baking sheet with parchment paper.
2. Wash and dry the tomatoes, and halve them crosswise. Put them cut-side up on the parchment paper, and drizzle them with ¼ cup of olive oil, allowing the oil to pool on the parchment paper. Sprinkle with the salt and pepper.

3. Roast for 3 to 4 hours, or until the edges of the tomatoes are puckered and the cut surface is a little dry.

4. Sprinkle with the balsamic vinegar and let cool on the baking sheet.

5. Pack into an airtight container, and pour any excess oil from the parchment paper on top. Add the remaining 1 tablespoon of oil to the container. Seal and refrigerate for up to one month.

Nutrition: Calories: 123 Fat: 12g Carbs: 5g Protein: 1g

Crispy Spicy Chickpeas

Preparation Time: 5 minutes

Cooking Time: 30 minutes

Servings: 1

Ingredients:

- 1 cup canned chickpeas, drained and rinsed
- 1 tablespoon olive oil
- ½ teaspoon kosher salt
- ⅛ Teaspoon freshly ground black pepper
- ½ teaspoon smoked paprika
- ⅛ Teaspoon cayenne pepper

Directions:

1. Preheat the oven to 400°F.
2. Remove any remaining moisture from the chickpeas by rolling them between two paper towels. Place in a medium bowl.
3. Add the olive oil, salt, and pepper to the bowl and toss to completely coat the chickpeas.
4. Spread them out on a baking sheet. Roast for 20 minutes, stir, and roast for an additional 10 minutes, or until lightly crisped.

5. When it's still warm, toss the chickpeas with the smoked paprika and cayenne pepper. Adding the spices last prevents them from charring in the oven and provides a crispier chickpea.

6. You can keep at a room temperature in an open container for several days. This keeps them crisper longer, although they'll start to lose some crispness over time. They can also be stored in the refrigerator once they've completely cooled.

Nutrition: Calories: 101 Fat: 4g Carbs: 14g Protein: 3g

Roasted Pumpkin Seeds

Preparation Time: 5 minutes

Cooking Time: 10 minutes

Servings: 1

Ingredients:

- 1 cup unsalted pumpkin seeds
- 1 teaspoon olive oil
- ¼ teaspoon kosher salt
- Pinch cayenne pepper
- Pinch smoked paprika

Directions:

1. Using a small bowl, combine all of the ingredients.
2. Heat a small sauté pan over medium-low heat. Add the pumpkin seeds and sauté, tossing frequently as they brown, for 10 minutes, or until they reach your preferred level of toasting.
3. Cool and store at room temperature in an airtight container for up to two months or in the refrigerator for up to one year.

Nutrition: Calories: 20 Fat: 1g Carbs: 2g Protein: 1g

Lemony Breadcrumbs

Preparation Time: 5 minutes

Cooking Time: 10 minutes

Servings: 1

Ingredients:

- 2 teaspoons olive oil
- 1 cup panko
- ⅛ Teaspoon kosher salt
- ⅛ Teaspoon freshly ground black pepper
- Zest of 1 lemon (about ½ teaspoon or more, to taste)

Directions:

1. Using a small skillet over a medium heat, warm the olive oil. Add the panko, salt, and pepper. Toss to lightly coat, and toast until the breadcrumbs are a golden color, about 3 minutes. You'll need to stir the breadcrumbs about every 30 seconds so they toast evenly.

2. Take it out from the heat, and stir in the lemon zest.

3. Transfer to a plate to cool before storing in an airtight container.

Nutrition: Calories: 63 Fat: 2g Carbs: 10g Protein: 2g

Cauliflower Skillet Steaks

Preparation Time: 15 minutes

Cooking Time: 15 minutes

Servings: 4

Ingredients:

- 1 large head cauliflower, sliced into 6 (1-inch-thick) steaks
- 2 tablespoons olive oil, divided
- ½ teaspoon smoked paprika
- ½ teaspoon kosher salt
- ¼ teaspoon cayenne pepper
- Balsamic Roasted Tomatoes

Directions:

1. Rub both sides of the cauliflower steaks lightly with 1 tablespoon of olive oil, and sprinkle on both sides with the paprika, salt, and cayenne.
2. Heat the remaining 1 tablespoon of olive oil in a large sauté pan over medium-high heat. Arrange the cauliflower steaks in the pan, including any extra florets. You need to cook the steaks in two batches.

3. Cook the cauliflower until slightly crisped, about 3 minutes per side. Reduce the heat to medium and continue to cook for another 8 to 10 minutes, or until the cauliflower is tender when pierced with a sharp knife.
4. Serve the cauliflower steaks topped with the roasted tomatoes.

Nutrition: Calories: 114 Fat: 8g Carbs: 11g Protein: 4g

Lemony Kale, Avocado, and Chickpea Salad

Preparation Time: 20 minutes

Cooking Time: 0 minute

Servings: 4

Ingredients:

- 1 avocado, halved
- 2 tablespoons freshly squeezed lemon juice, divided
- ½ teaspoon kosher salt, divided
- 1 bunch curly kale, stems removed and discarded, leaves coarsely chopped (about 8 cups)
- 1 (15-ounce) can chickpeas, drained and rinsed
- 2 tablespoons extra-virgin olive oil
- ¼ teaspoon freshly ground black pepper
- ¼ cup Roasted Pumpkin Seeds or store-bought

Direction:

1. Slice your avocado then coop its flesh from one of the avocado halves out of its skin and put it in a large bowl. Put a 1 tablespoon of lemon juice

and ¼ teaspoon of salt, and mash everything together. Add the coarsely chopped kale leaves and massage them by hand with the avocado mash until the kale becomes tender. Place the kale-avocado mash on a serving plate.

2. Remove the flesh of the remaining avocado half from its skin and chop into bite-size chunks. Place in the bowl that contained the kale, and add the chickpeas.

3. In a small bowl, whisk together the olive oil, remaining 1 tablespoon of lemon juice, remaining ¼ teaspoon of salt, and the pepper. Drizzle over the chickpeas and avocado and toss to combine. Pile on top of the kale-avocado mash, and top with the roasted pumpkin seeds.

Nutrition: Calories: 383 Fat: 20g Carbs: 43g Protein: 14g

Lentil Potato Salad

Preparation Time: 10 minutes

Cooking Time: 25 minutes

Servings: 2

Ingredients:

- ½ cup beluga lentils
- 8 fingerling potatoes
- 1 cup thinly sliced scallions
- ¼ cup halved cherry tomatoes
- ¼ cup Lemon Vinaigrette
- Kosher salt, to taste
- Freshly ground black pepper, to taste

Directions:

1. Pour 2 cups of water to simmer in a small pot and add the lentils. Cover and simmer for 20 to 25 minutes, or until the lentils are tender. Drain and set aside to cool.

2. While the lentils are cooking, bring a medium pot of well-salted water to a boil and add the potatoes. Low heat to simmer and cook for about 15 minutes, or until the potatoes are

tender. Drain. Once cool enough to handle, slice or halve the potatoes.

3. Place the lentils on a serving plate and top with the potatoes, scallions, and tomatoes. Drizzle with the vinaigrette and season with the salt and pepper.

Nutrition: Calories: 400 Fat: 26g Carbs: 39g Protein: 7g

Curried Apple Chips

Preparation Time: 15 minutes

Cooking Time: 1 hour and 30 minutes

Servings: 25 chips

Ingredients:

- 1 tablespoon freshly squeezed lemon juice
- ½ cup water
- 2 apples, such as Fuji or Honey crisp, cored and thinly sliced into rings
- 1 teaspoon curry powder

Directions:

1. Preheat the oven to 200°F.Put a rimmed baking sheet with parchment paper.
2. Mix the lemon juice and water together in a medium bowl. As soon as the apples are sliced, add them to the bowl to soak for 2 minutes. Drain and pat dry with paper towels. Arrange in a single layer on the baking sheet.
3. Place the curry powder in a sieve or other sifter and lightly sprinkle the apple slices. Not too

much curry goes a long way, so it's is okay not to dust both side of the apple rings.

4. In you preheated oven bake it for 45 minutes. After 45 minutes, turn the slices over and bake for another 45 minutes, again without opening the oven. If you find the apple chips need additional crisping, bake for another 15 minutes.

5. For the crispiest texture, let the chips cool before eating, but they're pretty fabulous slightly warm.

Nutrition: Calories: 61 Fat: 0g Carbs: 16g Protein: 0g

Bok Choy–Asparagus Salad

Preparation Time: 20 minutes

Cooking Time: 0 minute

Servings: 4

Ingredients:

- 4 cups coarsely chopped baby bok Choy
- 1½ cups asparagus, trimmed and cut into 1½-inch lengths
- 1 cup cauliflower rice
- 1 cup strawberries, chopped into bite-size chunks
- 1 mango, peeled and diced
- ½ cup scallions, sliced into 1-inch lengths
- ¼ cup Lemon Vinaigrette

Directions:

1. In a large bowl, combine the bok choy, asparagus, cauliflower rice, strawberries, mango, and scallions. Drizzle with the vinaigrette and gently toss.

Nutrition: Calories: 210 Fat: 14g Carbs: 21g Protein: 3g

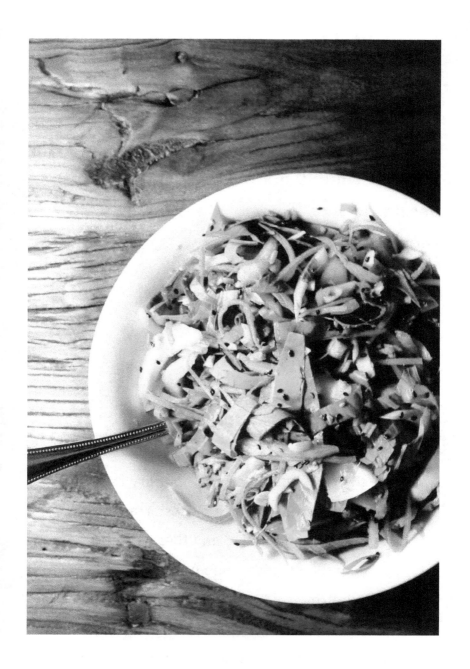

Lemony Romaine and Avocado Salad

Preparation Time: 15 minutes

Cooking Time: 0 minute

Servings: 6

Ingredients:

- 1 head romaine lettuce
- ½ cup pomegranate seeds
- ¼ cup pine nuts
- ¼ cup Lemon Vinaigrette
- 2 avocados
- Freshly ground black pepper

Directions:

2. Wash your vegetables and spin-dry then slice the leaves into bite-size pieces. Transfer the leaves in a large bowl, and toss with the pomegranate seeds, pine nuts, and half of the vinaigrette.

3. Slice the avocados in half. Remove the pit from each, and slice the avocados into long thin

slices. Using a large spoon, carefully scoop the slices out of the peel.

4. Arrange your avocado slices on top of the lettuce in the bowl, and drizzle half of the remaining dressing over them. Carefully toss using your hands or a large metal spoon. Add the remaining dressing as needed.

5. Finish with a few sprinkles of pepper.

Nutrition: Calories: 217 Fat: 20g Carbs: 11g Protein 3g

Strawberry-Coconut Smoothie

Preparation Time: 10 minutes

Cooking Time: 0 minute

Servings: 1

Ingredients:

- Dairy-free and Vegan: Use coconut milk yogurt
- 1 cup frozen strawberries, slightly thawed
- 1 very ripe banana, sliced and frozen
- ½ cup light coconut milk
- ½ cup plain Greek yogurt
- 1 teaspoon freshly squeezed lime juice
- 1 tablespoon chia seeds (optional)
- 3 or 4 ice cubes

Directions:

1. Transfer all your ingredients in a blender and blend until smooth. If necessary, add additional coconut milk or water to thin the smoothie to your preferred consistency.

Nutrition: Calories: 278 Fat: 2g Carbs: 57g Protein: 14g

Aloha Mango-Pineapple Smoothie

Preparation Time: 10 minutes

Cooking Time: 0 minute

Servings: 2

Ingredients:

- 1 large navel orange, peeled and quartered
- 1 cup frozen pineapple chunks
- 1 cup frozen mango chunks
- 1 tablespoon freshly squeezed lime juice
- ½ cup plain Greek yogurt
- ½ cup milk or coconut milk
- 1 tablespoon chia seeds (optional)
- 3 or 4 ice cubes

Directions:

1. Transfer all your ingredients in a blender and blend until smooth. If necessary, add additional milk or water to thin the smoothie to your preferred consistency.

Nutrition: Calories: 158 Fat: 1g Carbs: 35g Protein: 7g

Delicious Lentil Soup

Preparation Time: 15 Minutes

Cooking Time: 25 Minutes

Servings: 4

Ingredients:

- 1 tbsp. Olive Oil
- 4 cups Vegetable Stock
- 1 Onion, finely chopped
- 2 Carrots, medium
- 1 cup Lentils, dried
- 1 tsp. Cumin

Directions:

1. To make this healthy soup, first, you need to heat the oil in a medium-sized skillet over medium heat.
2. Once the oil becomes hot, stir in the cumin and then the onions.
3. Sauté those for 3 minutes or until the onion is slightly transparent and cooked.
4. To this, add the carrots and toss them well.
5. Next, stir in the lentils. Mix well.

6. Now, pour in the vegetable stock and give a good stir until everything comes together.
7. As the soup mixture starts to boil, reduce the heat and allow it to simmer for 10 minutes while keeping the pan covered.
8. Turn off the heat and then transfer the mixture to a bowl.
9. Finally, blend it with an immersion blender or in a high-speed blender for 1 minute or until you get a rich, smooth mixture.
10. Serve it hot and enjoy.

Nutrition: Calories: 251 Kcal Protein: 14g Carbohydrates: 41.3g Fat: 4.1g

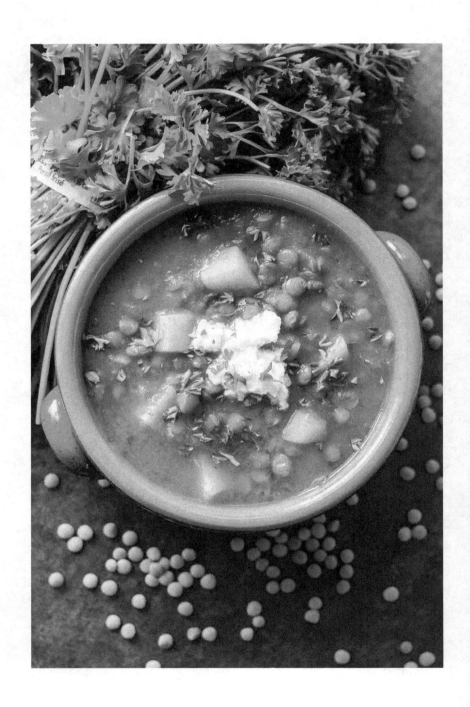

Trail Mix

Preparation Time: 10 Minutes

Cooking Time: 10 Minutes

Servings: 2

Ingredients:

- 1 cup Walnuts, raw
- 2 cups Tart Cherries, dried
- 1 cup Pumpkin Seeds, raw
- 1 cup Almonds, raw
- ½ cup Vegan Dark Chocolate
- 1 cup Cashew

Directions:

1. First, mix all the ingredients needed to make the trail mix in a large mixing bowl until combined well.
2. Store in an air-tight container.

Nutrition: Calories: 596 Kcal Protein: 17.5g Carbohydrates: 46.1g Fat: 39.5g

Flax Crackers

Preparation Time: 5 Minutes

Cooking Time: 60 Minutes

Servings: 4 to 6

Ingredients:

- 1 cup Flaxseeds, whole
- 2 cups Water
- ¾ cup Flaxseeds, grounded
- 1 tsp. Sea Salt
- ½ cup Chia Seeds
- 1 tsp. Black Pepper
- ½ cup Sunflower Seeds

Directions:

1. Using a large bowl, you need to put all your ingredients then mix them well. Soak them in a water for about 10 to 15 minutes.
2. After that, transfer the mixture to a parchment paper-lined baking sheet and spread it evenly. Tip: Make sure the paper lines the edges as well.
3. Next, bake it for 60 minutes at 350 °F.

4. Once the time is up, flip the entire bar and take off the parchment paper.

5. Bake for half an hour or until it becomes crispy and browned.

6. Allow it to cool completely and then break it down.

Nutrition: Calories: 251cal Proteins: 9.2g Carbohydrates: 14.9g Fat: 16g

Crunchy Granola

Preparation Time: 10 Minutes

Cooking Time: 20 Minutes

Servings: 1

Ingredients:

- ½ cup Oats
- Dash of Salt
- 2 tbsp. Vegetable Oil
- 3 tbsp. Maple Syrup
- 1/3 cup Apple Cider Vinegar
- ½ cup Almonds
- 1 tsp. Cardamom, grounded

Directions:

1. Preheat the oven to 375 °F.
2. After that, mix oats, pistachios, salt, and cardamom in a large bowl.
3. Next, spoon in the vegetable oil and maple syrup to the mixture.
4. Then, transfer the mixture to a parchment-paper-lined baking sheet.

5. Bake them for 13 minutes or until the mixture is toasted. Tip: Check on them now and then. Spread it out well.

6. Return the sheet to the oven for further ten minutes.

7. From your oven remove the sheet and allow it to cool completely.

8. Serve and enjoy.

Nutrition: Calories: 763Kcal Proteins: 12.9g Carbohydrates: 64.8g Fat: 52.4g

Chickpea Scramble Bowl

Preparation Time: 10 Minutes

Cooking Time: 10 Minutes

Servings: Makes 2 Bowl

Ingredients:

- ¼ of 1 Onion, diced
- 15 oz. Chickpeas
- 2 Garlic cloves, minced
- ½ tsp. Turmeric
- ½ tsp. Black Pepper
- ½ tsp. Extra Virgin Olive Oil
- ½ tsp. Salt

Directions:

1. Begin by placing the chickpeas in a large bowl along with a bit of water.
2. Soak for few minutes and then mash the chickpeas lightly with a fork while leaving some of them in the whole form.
3. Next, spoon in the turmeric, pepper, and salt to the bowl. Mix well.

4. Then, heat oil in a medium-sized skillet over medium-high heat.

5. Once the oil becomes hot, stir in the onions.

6. Sauté the onions for 3 to 4 minutes or until softened.

7. Then, add the garlic and cook for further 1 minute or until aromatic.

8. After that, stir in the mashed chickpeas. Cook for another 4 minutes or until thickened.

9. Serve along with micro greens. Place the greens at the bottom, followed by the scramble, and top it with cilantro or parsley.

Nutrition: Calories: 801Kcal Proteins: 41.5g Carbohydrates: 131.6g Fat: 14.7g

Maple Flavored Oatmeal

Preparation Time: 5 Minutes

Cooking Time: 25 Minutes

Servings: 2

Ingredients:

- 2 tbsp. Maple Syrup
- 1 cup Oatmeal
- ½ tsp. Cinnamon
- 2 ½ cup Water
- 2/3 cup Soy Milk
- 1 tsp. Earth Balance or Vegan Butter

Directions:

1. To start with, place oatmeal and water in a medium-sized saucepan over medium-high heat.
2. Bring the mixture to a boil.
3. Next, lower the heat and cook for further 13 to 15 minutes while keeping the pan covered. Tip: At this point, all the water should get absorbed by the grains.

4. Now, remove the pan from the heat and fluff this mixture with a fork.
5. Cover the pan again. Set it aside for 5 minutes.
6. Then, stir in all the remaining ingredients to the oatmeal mixture until everything comes together.
7. Serve and enjoy.

Nutrition: Calories: 411Kcal Proteins: 14.7g Carbohydrates: 73.6g Fat: 6.6g

Protein Pancakes

Preparation Time: 5 Minutes

Cooking Time: 10 Minutes

Servings: Makes 6 Pancakes

Ingredients:

- 1 cup All-Purpose Flour
- 2 tbsp. Maple Syrup
- ¼ cup Brown Rice Protein Powder
- ½ tsp. Sea Salt
- 1 tbsp. Baking Powder
- 1 cup Water

Directions:

1. To make these delightful protein-rich pancakes, you first need to combine the flour, sea salt, baking powder, and vegan protein powder in a large mixing bowl.
2. Spoon in the maple syrup and then later gradually add the water until you get a thick and lumpy batter.
3. Now, heat a non-stick pan over medium-high heat.

4. Then, scoop a ladle of the batter into it and cook the pancakes for 2 to 3 minutes or until bubbles form.

5. Cook each side for a further minute.

6. Serve immediately.

Nutrition: Calories: 295 Kcal Protein: 15.8g Carbohydrates: 59.9g Fat: 1.2g

Squash Lentil Soup

Preparation Time: 10 Minutes

Cooking Time: 35 Minutes

Servings: 4

Ingredients:

- 7 cups Vegetable Broth
- 2 tbsp. Olive Oil
- 2 tsp., Sage dried
- 1 Yellow Onion, medium & diced.
- Salt & Pepper t0 taste
- 1 Butternut Squash
- 1 ½ cup Red Lentils

Directions:

1. Using a saucepan start heating your oil, and stir in the onions.
2. Sauté the onions for to 2 to 3 minutes or until softened.
3. Once cooked, stir in squash and sage while stirring continuously.
4. Then, spoon in the lentils, salt, and pepper.

5. Bring the lentil mixture to a boil for about 30 minutes. Lower the heat.

6. Then, allow the soup to cool down until the lentils are soft.

7. Finally, transfer the mixture to a high-speed blender and blend for 3 to 4 minutes or until smooth.

8. Serve hot.

Nutrition: Calories: 421 Kcal Protein: 16.7g Carbohydrates: 51g Fat: 4.5g

Sweet Potato Gnocchi

Preparation Time: 30 minutes

Cooking Time: 30 minutes

Servings: 2

Ingredients

- 2 cups flour
- ¼ teaspoon salt
- ½ teaspoon turmeric
- 3 garlic cloves, roasted
- 1 sweet potato

Directions

1. To begin this recipe, you will want to heat your oven to 375°f. Once the oven is warm, place the sweet potato on a baking sheet and pop it in for thirty minutes.

2. During the last five minutes of the bake time, add the garlic cloves into the oven and allow them to roast.

3. When the time is up, remove the baking sheet from the oven and allow the ingredients to cool for ten minutes or so.

4. Next, you will want to remove the skin of the sweet potato. Once this is done, place the sweet potato into a mixing bowl and add in the garlic. Carefully take a fork and mash everything together until there are no chunks.

5. At this point, you can season the sweet potato with the turmeric and salt.

6. With the sweet potato now seasoned, it is time to add the flour. You will want to add the flour in a half of a cup at a time.

7. Be sure to stir the ingredients together well before you add any more flour in. The amount of flour may vary depending on the size of the sweet potato. You will want to continue adding flour until it becomes difficult to stir.

8. Now, your sweet potato should have a dough-like consistency. Break the dough up and roll the sweet potato into strips.

9. Using a knife, you can cut these strips into half-inch pieces.

10. Once you have finished making your gnocchi, you will want to take a large pot of water and bring it to a boil over high heat.

11. When your water is boiling carefully drop in the gnocchi pieces.

12. When they are cooked through, the pieces will rise to the top. Typically, this will take two to three minutes. Enjoy!

Nutrition: Calories: 460 Fat: 5 g Carbs: 45 g Protein: 10 g

Taco Pasta Bowl

Preparation Time: 10 minutes

Cooking Time: 30 minutes

Servings: 4

Ingredients:

- 1 can black beans
- 1 cup corn
- ½ cup diced onion
- 1 jar salsa
- 1 box pasta
- ¼ teaspoon cumin
- 2 tablespoons chili powder

Directions:

1. To start, please cook the pasta of your choice according to the directions provided on the box. Once this step is complete, you can drain the water and set the pasta to the side.

2. Next, you will want to take a medium pan and place it over medium to high heat. Add one tablespoon of your oil and bring it to sizzle. Once the oil is hot, place your onion and cook for

three to five minutes. By the end, the onion should be soft.

3. At this point, you will add in the beans, corn, salsa, and spices. I have chosen to use chili powder and cumin, but you can spice your dish however you would like!

4. Last, you will pour your sauce over your pasta and enjoy!

Nutrition: Calories: 480 Fat: 8 g Carbs: 46 g Protein: 18 g

Vegan BBQ Tofu

Preparation Time: 10 minutes

Cooking Time: 40 minutes

Servings: 3

Ingredients:

- ¼ cup vegan BBQ sauce
- ¼ teaspoon pepper
- ¼ teaspoon garlic powder
- ¼ teaspoon salt
- 1 tablespoon grape seed oil
- 1 pack firm tofu

Directions:

1. Before you begin cooking your tofu, you will want to press it. Generally, this will take thirty to forty-five minutes. If possible, try to press the tofu overnight so that it is ready for you when you need it.

2. Once your tofu is ready, bring a saucepan over medium heat and allow it to warm up. As your saucepan is warming up, slice your tofu into small pieces. Put a 1 tablespoon of oil and

spread your tofu across the pan. At this point, season your tofu and cook for five minutes. Be sure to flip each piece of tofu until it is a nice golden-brown colour all over.

3. Finally, remove the tofu from the pan and cover it in BBQ sauce. This meal is excellent alone or with your favorite grain or vegetable.

Nutrition: Calories: 290, Fat: 64 g, Carbs: 25 g, Protein: 20 g

Mustard Tomato Mix

Preparation time: 10 minutes

Cooking time: 10 minutes

Servings: 4

Ingredients:

- 2 pounds plum tomatoes, sliced
- A pinch of salt and black pepper
- 2 tablespoons avocado oil
- 3 tablespoons lime juice
- 1 tablespoon Dijon mustard
- 1 tablespoon mint, chopped

Directions:

1. Using a pan heat your oil over medium heat, add the tomatoes, the lime juice and the other ingredients, toss, cook for 10 minutes, divide between plates and serve.

Nutrition: Calories: 120 Fat: 4 g Carbs: 15 g Protein: 6 g

Veggies and noodle bowl with mushrooms

Preparation Time: 10 minutes

Cooking Time: 20 minutes

Servings: 2

Ingredients:

- 8 ounces sliced mushrooms
- 9 oz. rinsed and sliced leeks
- 8 ounces noodles
- 5 ounces baby spinach

Directions:

1. Boil the noodles according to the given directions on the packet, remove the boiling water, rinse with cold water, and set aside.
2. Now take a bowl, add all the ingredients, and whisk them well until all the ingredients are combined well.

Nutrition: Calories: 260 Fat: 4 g Carbs: 35 g Protein: 4 g

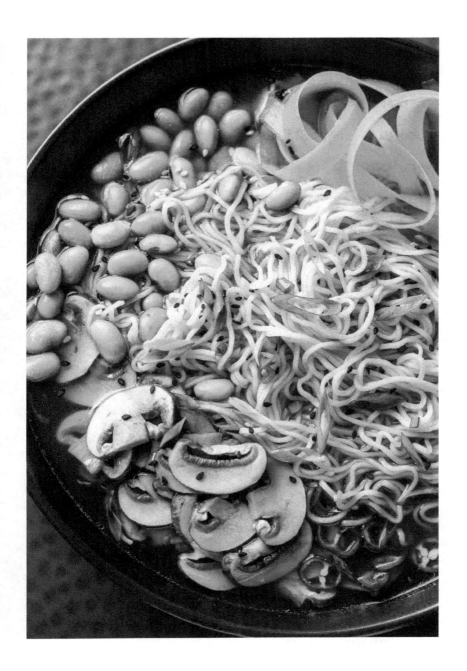

Broccoli over Orzo

Preparation Time: 10 minutes

Cooking Time: 25 minutes

Servings: 3

Ingredients:

- 3 teaspoons olive oil
- 4 garlic cloves, smashed
- 2 cups broccoli florets
- 4½ ounces orzo pasta
- ¼ teaspoon salt
- ¼ teaspoon pepper

Directions:

1. Start off by preparing your broccoli. You can do this by trimming the stems off and slicing the broccoli into small, bite-size pieces. If you want, go ahead and season with salt.

2. Next, you will want to steam your broccoli over a little bit of water until it is cooked through. Once the broccoli is cooked, chop it up into even smaller pieces.

3. When the broccoli is done, cook your pasta according to the directions provided on the box. Once this is done, drain the water and then place the pasta back into the pot.

4. With the pasta and broccoli done, place it back into the pot with the garlic. Stir everything together well and cook until the garlic turns a nice golden colour. Be sure to stir everything to combine your meal well. Serve warm and enjoy a simple dinner!

Nutrition: Calories: 310 Fat: 4 g Carbs: 35 g Protein: 10 g

Mango Pineapple Hoisin Sauce

Preparation Time: 10 minutes

Cooking Time: 10 minutes

Servings: 2

Ingredients:

- 1 ½ cups fresh mango juice or pureed mango
- ⅔ cup vegan hoisin sauce
- 4 tablespoons brown rice vinegar
- 1 cup fresh pineapple juice
- ½ cup tamari or soy sauce
- 2 tablespoons Sriracha sauce

Directions:

1. Use a pan and heat oil over medium heat.
2. Add all the ingredients and stir constantly.
3. Simmer until the mixture thickens.

Nutrition: Calories: 125 Fat: 2 g Carbs: 8 g
Protein: 4.3 g

Sriracha Sauce

Preparation Time: 20 minutes

Cooking Time: 10 minutes

Servings: 2

Ingredients

- 15 red Fresno chilies, chopped into chunks
- ½ tablespoon salt
- 4 garlic cloves
- ¼ cup apple cider or white vinegar
- 2 tablespoons raw sugar

Directions:

1. Place the chilies, garlic, salt and sugar into a food processor. Pulse until coarsely chopped. Transfer into a mason's jar.
2. Cover with a plastic cling and leave it for 5-7 days to ferment. Stir often during this period. In 3-4 days you will see some bubbles appearing.
3. Transfer the contents of the jar into a blender. Add vinegar and blend until smooth.
4. Transfer into a saucepan after passing through a wire mesh strainer.

5. Bring to a boil on high heat.

6. When it starts boiling, reduce the heat and simmer for 5 minutes. Remove from heat and cool.

7. Transfer into a flip top bottle. Refrigerate until use.

Nutrition: Calories: 90 Fat: 6 g Carbs: 5 g Protein: 1 g

White Sauce (Béchamel)

Preparation Time: 10 minutes

Cooking Time: 12 minutes

Servings: 2

Ingredients:

- 6 tablespoons olive oil
- 4 cups soymilk or any other non-dairy milk of your choice
- 5 tablespoons all-purpose flour
- Sea salt to taste
- Black pepper to taste

Directions:

1. Place a heavy pot over a medium heat. Add oil. When the oil is heated, add sifted flour into the pan. Stir constantly for about a minute. It will begin to change color; be careful not to burn it!
2. Pour in the milk, stirring constantly. Keep stirring until thick.
3. Simmer until the thickness you desire is nearly achieved. This is because the sauce thickens further as it cools.

4. Turn off the heat. Add salt, pepper and any other herbs and spices if you desire.

Nutrition: Calories: 68 Fat: 2 g Carbs: 1.5 g Protein: 5 g

Conclusion

Vegan recipes do not need to be boring. There are so many different combinations of veggies, fruits, whole grains, beans, seeds, and nuts that you will be able to make unique meal plans for many months. These recipes contain the instructions along with the necessary ingredients and nutritional information.

If you ever come across someone complaining that they can't follow the plant-based diet because it's expensive, hard to cater for, lacking in variety, or tasteless, feel free to have them take a look at this book. In no time, you'll have another companion walking beside you on this road to healthier eating and better living.

Although healthy, many people are still hesitant to give vegan food a try. They mistakenly believe that these would be boring, tasteless, and complicated to make. This is the farthest thing from the truth.

Fruits and vegetables are organically delicious, fragrant, and vibrantly colored. If you add herbs, mushrooms, and nuts to the mix, dishes will always come out packed full of flavor it only takes a bit of effort and time to prepare great-tasting vegan meals for your family.

How easy was that? Don't we all want a seamless and easy way to cook like this?

I believe cooking is taking a better turn and the days, when we needed so many ingredients to provide a decent meal, were gone. Now, with easy tweaks, we can make delicious, quick, and easy meals. Most importantly, we get to save a bunch of cash on groceries.

I am grateful for downloading this book and taking the time to read it. I know that you have learned a lot and you had a great time reading it. Writing books is the best way to share the skills I have with your and the best tips too.

I know that there are many books and choosing my book is amazing. I am thankful that you stopped and took time to decide. You made a great decision and I am sure that you enjoyed it.

I will be even happier if you will add some comments. Feedbacks helped by growing and they still do. They help me to choose better content and new ideas. So, maybe your feedback can trigger an idea for my next book.

Hopefully, this book has helped you understand that vegetarian recipes and diet can improve your life, not only by improving your health and helping you lose weight, but also by saving you money and time. I sincerely hope that the recipes provided in this book have proven to be quick, easy, and delicious, and have provided you with enough variety to keep your taste buds interested and curious.

I hope you enjoyed reading about my book!

CPSIA information can be obtained
at www.ICGtesting.com
Printed in the USA
BVHW092237260421
605884BV00008B/156